© Franklin Watts 1988

Designed and produced by
Aladdin Books and David West
Children's Book Design
28 Percy Street
London W1P 5FF

First published in the
United States in 1988 by
Franklin Watts
387 Park Avenue South
New York, NY 10016

First Paperback Edition 1990

ISBN 0-531-10592-X (lib. bdg.)
ISBN 0-531-15211-1 (pbk.)

Library of Congress Catalog
Card Number: 88-50492

Printed in Belgium

This book is not intended as a substitute for the medical advice of physicians. The reader should consult a physician in matters relating to sexually transmitted diseases or other aspects of his or her health and particularly in respect to any symptoms that may require diagnosis or medical attention.

CONTENTS

TEEN · GUIDE · TO

SAFE SEX

Alan E. Nourse M.D.

Franklin Watts
New York · London · Toronto · Sydney

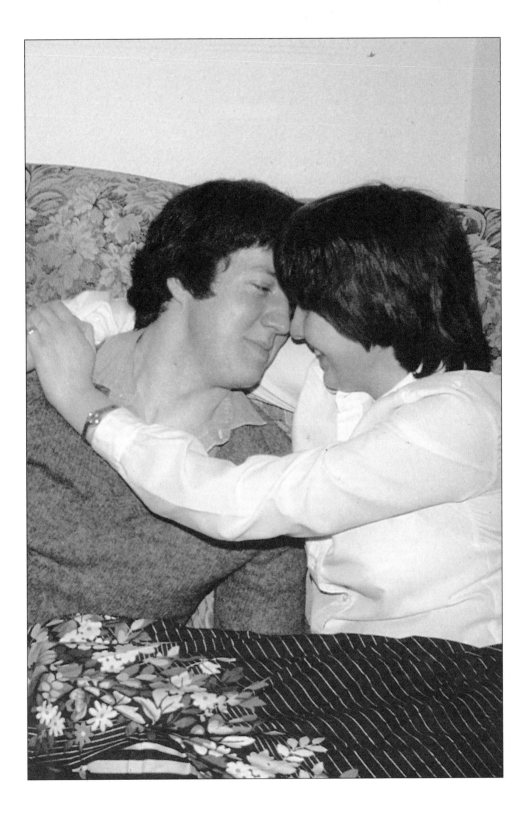

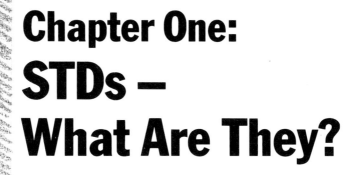

Chapter One:
STDs –
What Are They?

Although most people would rather not talk about STDs, it is important to know about them because these are the diseases that are passed from one person to another by sex contact.

More and more teenagers are beginning to suspect these days that having sex can be hazardous to their health. There are a number of very unpleasant and dangerous infections that can be passed from one person to another during sex. These are often called *sexually transmitted diseases*, or STDs for short. They can cause no end of trouble for the people who meet up with them.

This book is about these sexually transmitted diseases and how to keep from getting them by taking some common-sense measures called safe sex. You've probably heard of safe sex in connection with AIDS, one of the most dangerous of all the STDs. But safe sex can apply to all the other STDs as well. This book is about how you can protect yourself from these diseases if and when you *do* have sex.

Everybody knows what infections are. When you cut your finger, it may become sore and swollen; the cut has become infected by germs from the surface of your skin. You've all caught head colds or the flu. These are infections caused by germs that are breathed out by infected persons. And most people know about diarrhea – loose bowel movements – caused by germs growing in spoiled food. Infections of this sort are an ordinary fact of life. Everybody gets them now and then, and nobody is shy about talking about them.

Sexually transmitted diseases, or STDs, are different. These diseases are also infections, spread by different kinds of germs. But nobody likes to talk about them very much. The reason is that the germs of STDs are all passed from one person to another by sex contact, and most of them affect the sex organs directly. Not everybody gets these infections. You only get an STD by having sex – and then only if you're unlucky enough to have sex with someone who already has a sexually transmitted disease to pass on to you.

You may never even have heard of some of these infections. But it's very important that you know about them. Although some are just nuisances, others are really dangerous. Many can cause very unpleasant symptoms. Some of them can make serious trouble for you later, if they aren't discovered and treated early. Some can even cause death. And any one of them can upset your life very seriously.

Trouble with STDs

Sexually transmitted diseases can affect people's lives in many different ways, almost all of them bad. Consider the problems they caused for these four young people:

Just four months ago Gail T, age 14, started going steady with the most popular boy in her class. She thought it was great that a guy like Tom seemed to like her so much. They started having sex almost immediately. Everything was fine for a couple of months. But then Gail started to feel sick. She began having severe stomach pains and cramps. She started running a fever. Having sex began to hurt, and she seemed to have a lot of discharge all of a sudden. She didn't want to tell anybody about it, so she just toughed it out for a couple of months until her mom finally saw how sick she was and took her to a doctor.

Gail T. had an STD known as **gonorrhea**. Like many girls, she didn't have any noticeable symptoms at first. But soon the infection had spread from her vagina up into her Fallopian tubes. (There's more about the sex organs affected by STDs in the next chapter.) This caused swelling and soreness that her doctor called **pelvic inflammatory disease**, or **PID**. He ordered some antibiotic pills for Gail to take. In a few days the pain, cramps, and fever were gone. But Gail had to be checked from time to time to be sure the infection was completely cured.

Actually, Gail was very lucky that she got so sick and had to get help early. Sometimes a gonorrhea infection in a girl will just sit and smoulder for months and months without causing many symptoms at all. But during that time it can damage a girl's tubes so badly that she can never get pregnant later. This is a major cause of infertility – the inability to have a baby – in young women.

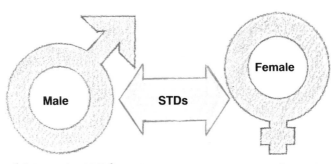

Sexually transmitted diseases can be caught by either the male or the female, so either male or female can pass them on to someone else. This means that neither sex alone is "to blame" for spreading STDs.

Greg H., at the age of 15, got in trouble with an STD during his summer vacation at the beach. He and his buddies met some girls cruising on the boardwalk one night and ended up having a great beach party. Greg never saw the girl again, but ten days later his hips began aching, and the next day he found a little cluster of very painful, itchy blisters on his penis.

Greg's father suspected the worst and took him to a doctor. A lab test showed that Greg had been infected with **genital herpes**. The doctor ordered a salve that helped quiet down the infection, but a month later it came back again. Greg then had to start taking some very expensive pills to help keep the infection from coming back. Of course, scientists know that genital herpes doesn't kill otherwise healthy young people, or cause any serious harm to the body. But it doesn't go away, either. For Greg, it will be a painful, embarrassing nuisance that may come back again and again for years. It will certainly interfere with his sex life in the future. The sad part is that Greg could have protected himself from this infection if he had known about it in time.

Josh W., age 22, has a far more serious problem. Just home from the Navy, he and Marcie planned to get married. But when Josh had a pre-marital physical exam with his family doctor, a blood test came back positive for **syphilis**. Marcie wasn't exactly pleased about this, and Josh was floored. True, he'd had sex with lots of different girls. But he'd never had any symptoms he could remember. (The early signs of syphilis, one of the most dangerous STDs, are often easily overlooked.) The truth is, Josh was very lucky this disease was detected when it was. This report may not help his wedding plans very much. But at least he has now been treated and cured of the infection. Without treatment, syphilis could have caused enormous damage to Josh's body and brain over the years. And it might very well finally have killed him.

At age 16, Kathy K. is suddenly terrified and doesn't know what to do.

She's known all along that the biker she's been riding with for the last year has been shooting up drugs. But now she's learned that one of his best buddies has AIDS. Kathy has heard that the AIDS virus is passed from one person to another on dirty needles – and that it's also passed on through sex. Could her biker boyfriend be infected? Could she? He won't go and have an AIDS test. Should she? She's read that not many girls get the AIDS virus this way. But some do. What if she's one of them? She can't talk to her folks about something like this. Who can she talk to? Suddenly Kathy is faced with some very serious and frightening questions – and she doesn't have any idea where to turn for help.

Knowing About STDs

These four young people have different problems. But they all have two things in common. All of them have been having sex, and all four have been exposed to sexually transmitted diseases. Unlike other infections, these diseases have a way of thoroughly messing up people's lives – sometimes permanently. What is more, STDs such as gonorrhea, syphilis, genital herpes, and chlamydia are now spreading more rapidly among teenagers than in any other age group. For one reason, more and more teenagers are having sex earlier today, so the risk of getting STDs is greater and greater for them. For another, very few young people know much about these diseases, or how to protect themselves from STD infections.

Your first line of defense against STDs is to *know that they exist*. In this book we'll talk about what they are, what causes them, what symptoms to watch for, and what to do if you think you might be infected. Then we'll see how to protect yourself against these infections. A good place to start is with the tiny troublemakers that cause these infections in the first place, and the sex organs that generally become infected.

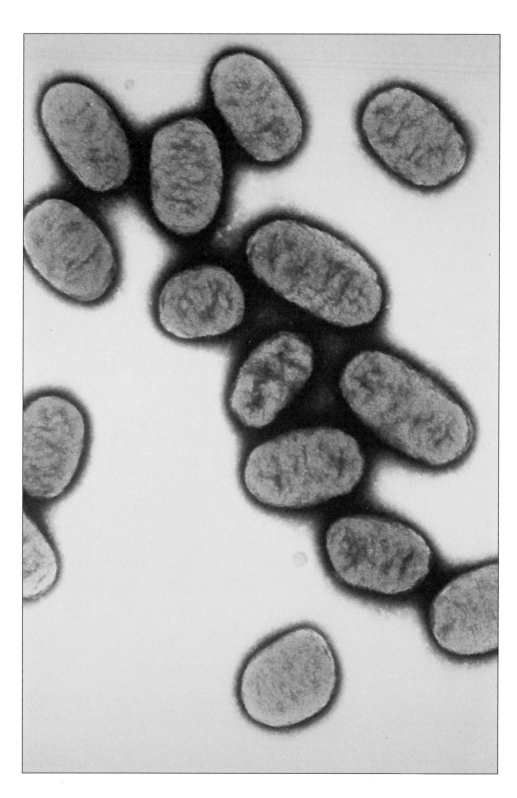

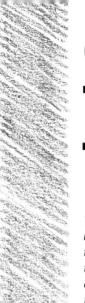

Chapter Two:
The Tiny
Troublemakers

Viruses are the simplest, most primitive of all living things. They are also the tiniest of all micro-organisms, so small that they can only be seen under an electron microscope.

Where do infections of any kind come from?

More than three hundred years ago a Dutch lens-grinder named Anton van Leeuwenhoek made a crude microscope by putting a finely ground magnifying lens into a tube. Peering at a drop of pond water through this tube, Leeuwenhoek made a remarkable discovery. He found that the drop was full of tiny living creatures far too small to see with the naked eye. Because some of these creatures seemed to move around on their own, he called them "animalcules" or "little animals."

Today we know that some of these "animalcules" are really tiny plants. Others are tiny animals. Still others seem to be somewhere in between. Scientists now call them all *micro-organisms* ("micro" means very small; an "organism" is any kind of a living creature). Most people just call them "germs."

Germs exist everywhere in the world. They live in our rivers, ponds, and oceans. They float in the air we breathe. They live on our skin, on the objects we touch, in our food, sometimes even inside our bodies.

Most micro-organisms are harmless to us. Many do good things, like the germs that decay rotting leaves and turn them into rich soil. But some, if they find their way into our bodies, can grow and multiply there and cause **infections**. These particular germs are called *pathogens*, or "disease-makers." There are several different kinds, and each kind causes trouble in a different way.

The Bacteria

The micro-organisms in one large group are called *bacteria*. These are tiny, one-celled plantlike organisms. They cannot be seen with the naked eye, but they're quite large, as micro-organisms go. Most can be seen under a microscope, especially when they have been colored or "stained" with a red or deep purple dye to make them show up.

Some bacteria are round or oval in shape. Doctors call these bacteria *cocci* (pronounced "COK-sigh"). *Streptococci*, or "strep," grow in long chains and cause severe throat infections. *Staphylococci*, or "staph," grow in clusters like grapes and cause pimples and other skin infections. *Diplo-cocci*, or "double cocci," grow in pairs. One kind can cause a dangerous in-fection of the spine and brain called *meningitis*. Another kind, called *gono-cocci*, live best on the warm, moist surfaces of the male or female sex organs. They are passed from one person to another during sex and cause a harmful sexually transmitted disease called **gonorrhea**.

Other bacteria can also cause STDs. Some, called *bacilli* (pronounced "buh-SIL-eye"), are shaped like rods. One group, known as *Ducrey's ba-cilli*, cause an uncommon STD called **chancroid infection**. Much more common is a very dangerous STD known as **syphilis**. This is caused by spiral-shaped bacilli called *spirochetes* ("SPY-rokeets"). They look like lit-tle corkscrews under the microscope. They are almost invisible because they won't soak up any dye to make them stand out. Doctors have to use

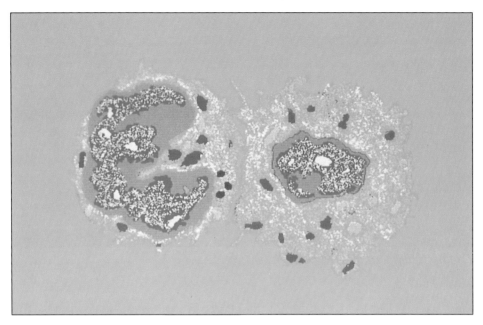

Gonococci under attack by white blood cells

special microscopes to see them at all. This can make syphilis hard to detect.

What do bacteria do that is so bad when they invade the body? First they begin damaging cells and tiny blood vessels in the area. To fight them off, the body sends in armies of special *white blood cells* to try to destroy them. The area where this battle is fought becomes swollen and sore, and the body temperature may rise. A *fever* usually means that an infection has started.

Sometimes the white blood cells win the battle. The bacteria are killed, and the body begins to heal the damage. This is what happens when a sore throat gets better after a few days even when you haven't taken anything for it. But often the bacteria aren't killed. The infection spreads. The germs may get into the bloodstream (sometimes called "blood poisoning") and spread to distant organs. There they continue to grow and multiply. This

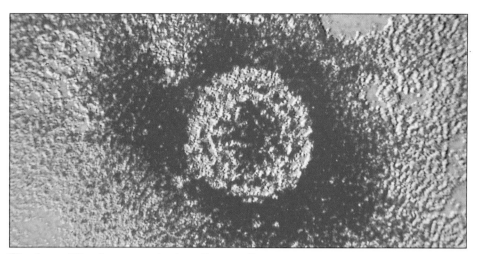

The hepatitis virus can destroy liver cells.

may sometimes lead to harmful infections in the lungs, the kidneys, the bones or joints, the brain, or other organs.

Before 1936 there wasn't much doctors could do to fight infections. Many people died of infectious diseases. Then a chemical called *sulfanilimide* was found. It prevented certain dangerous bacteria from growing. Within ten years drugs such as *penicillin* and *streptomycin* were discovered. They actually killed bacteria and cured many infections. They were called *antibiotics*. Today there are dozens of antibiotics to cure dangerous infections. Fortunately, some antibiotics will kill the bacteria that cause STDs such as gonorrhea or syphilis. But for treatment to be successful, these infections must be discovered and treated early, before too much damage has been done.

The Viruses

Viruses are a completely different kind of germ. They are the tiniest of all micro-organisms. They are so small they can't be seen under an ordinary microscope. Scientists can only see them with an electron microscope.

Viruses are also the simplest, most primitive of all living things. Some scientists wonder if they are really "living" at all. A virus is nothing more than a tiny bit of hereditary material called DNA or RNA, wrapped up in a protective envelope. Viruses can't multiply on their own, the way bacteria or other micro-organisms do. All a virus can do is make its way inside the living cells of some other creature, and then force those cells to make more viruses.

All the viruses we know are *parasites*. That means they make other creatures keep them alive, and don't do anything good in return. When they invade or infect other living cells they don't just make those cells produce more viruses. They usually kill the cells in the process. Then the newly made viruses go on to invade and kill other cells. The more viruses that are made, the more cells are killed. So when a disease-causing virus invades a human being, it can often cause a bad infection. A flu virus, for instance, can destroy cells in the lungs and cause *pneumonia*, sometimes severe enough to kill a person. A hepatitis virus can destroy cells in the liver and cause death from liver failure.

Fortunately, the human body can fight off most virus infections before they become deadly. The body's natural *immune system* (a complicated army of protective cells and chemicals) can often search out and destroy viruses. In many cases, the body's immune system remains alert after the virus is beaten off, so it can't come back and start another infection later. But other viruses hide from the body's immune system and never go away once they've gotten into the body.

Viruses cause many kinds of infections in people. Head colds, flu, measles, mumps, and chicken pox are all virus infections. And viruses can cause sexually transmitted diseases too. One STD caused by a virus is called genital herpes. Another is known as **AIDS**.

So far there are no antibiotic drugs to kill viruses. The best we have are a few drugs which slow down the production of new viruses inside the invaded cells. This means that diseases like genital herpes or AIDS are not curable. Sometime in the future genital herpes or AIDS may be prevented by vaccination shots, the way measles and mumps are today. But so far no vaccine has been found to prevent either of these infections.

Other Troublemakers

There are a few other kinds of germs that can also cause STDs. **Protozoans**, for example, are tiny one-celled animal-like organisms. One protozoan named **trichomonas** can cause an infection in the vagina. It can also infect the penis. It is sometimes passed back and forth between two people who have sex frequently. This can make the infection very hard to get rid of.

Various **yeasts**, a kind of fungus, can also cause vaginal infections and be transmitted to a sex partner. So can another germ, known as **chlamydia**. This is believed to be the most common and fast-spreading STD in the United States today. Fortunately, all these STDs can be treated and cured with the proper medicines once they have been detected.

The Target Organs

For most STDs, the sex organs themselves are the first targets of infection. Before we discuss individual STDs, we need to review those target organs most likely to be hit by sexually transmitted infections.

Most of a male's sex organs are located outside the body. The **penis** is a tube-shaped organ between the legs. When a male is excited about sex, his penis temporarily enlarges and becomes stiff with an **erection**. Behind the penis is a pouch of skin called the **scrotum** holding two oval sex glands, the **testicles**. They produce the sperm cells. Hollow tubes then carry the sperm up into the **pelvis** (the lowest part of the abdomen) for storage. During sex the sperm empty into the man's urine tube, called the **urethra**. This tube carries the sperm down the whole length of the penis to the outside. In the male most STD germs are likely to infect the penis first, or find their way up into the urethra and start the infection there.

A girl's sex organs are all inside her body except for the external entry to the vagina, which is called the **vulva**. The **vagina** is a stretchable internal tube or canal a few inches long connecting the vulva with the lower end of the **uterus**, or womb. The uterus is shaped like a small pear, with a narrow lower end, called the **cervix**, and an upper part, the **body**. It has thick walls made of muscle with a hollow space inside. A very narrow canal passes up through the cervix from the vagina into the space inside the uterus. This means that STD germs can make their way up. At the top of the uterus the internal space connects with a narrow tube on either side, called **Fallopian tubes**. These tubes extend up to contact small glands on either side called **ovaries**. In order for a girl to get pregnant, an egg cell must pass down one of the Fallopian tubes from an ovary to the uterus. So it's important those tubes don't get blocked.

When a girl is first infected by an STD germ, the infection may start on the external folds, or **labia**, of the vulva, or in her urine tube, or **urethra**. But some infections first affect the vagina or cervix, where they are harder to detect. And later, STD germs may work their way up through the uterus to cause an internal infection and blockage in the Fallopian tubes, or around the ovaries. This can be a harmful complication of an STD in a girl.

Whatever the STD, it is important to detect the infection as early as possible. To do this you need to know some facts about the individual infections. In the following chapters we will see how the major STDs behave, what tell-tale symptoms can occur, and what can be done about them.

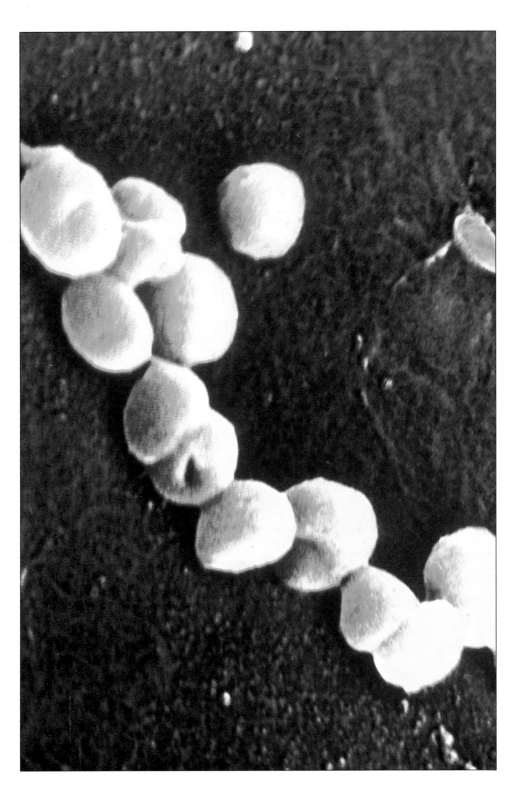

Chapter Three:
Gonorrhea and Syphilis

Some kinds of bacteria, micro-organisms so small they can only be seen under a microscope, can cause STDs. One of the most common bacteria-caused STDs is gonorrhea.

Two very different sexually transmitted diseases have been causing trouble for hundreds of years. They are called gonorrhea (pronounced "GON-oh-REE-uh") and syphilis ("SIF-i-lis"). Until the 1940s these infections were especially dangerous because there was no good treatment for either of them. Then antibiotic drugs were found that could cure both diseases. For a while doctors hoped that gonorrhea and syphilis would soon be wiped out. But no such thing happened. In fact, both infections are still extremely active today. And they are attacking teenagers and young people more than any other age group.

Gonorrhea

Everyone has heard of this disease. Sometimes it is called "clap," "a strain," "a dose," or "GC." With so many nicknames, you might guess that lots of people have trouble with this infection – and they do. Gonorrhea today is one of the most widespread of all STDs. Over 900,000 cases of gonorrhea were reported in the United States in 1986, and another 3,600,000 cases that same year *weren't* reported. Unfortunately, more than two thirds of these cases of gonorrhea are occurring in teenagers and young people.

Gonorrhea is primarily an infection of the urethra, or urine tube. In a woman, it can also infect the vagina, the cervix, the body of the uterus, and the Fallopian tubes. The infection is caused by small oval-shaped bacteria called *gonococci* that grow together in pairs like double coffee beans. (See photograph on page 18.)

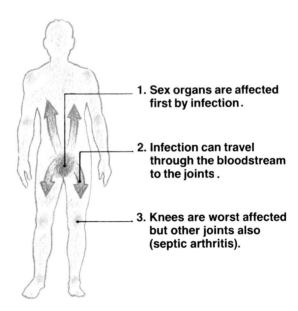

Gonorrhea first infects the sex organs – the urethra, *or* urine tube, in both sexes and the vagina *in the* female. If not treated, the infection can spread through the bloodstream to cause septic arthritis *in the knees, wrists, elbows, or other joints. In the female, the germs may also cause infection in the Fallopian tubes and ovaries, known as pelvic inflammatory disease, or PID, and can lead to infertility (inability to have a baby).*

1. **Sex organs are affected first by infection.**

2. **Infection can travel through the bloodstream to the joints.**

3. **Knees are worst affected but other joints also (septic arthritis).**

Gonococci are surprisingly weak, as bacteria go. They can live only a short time outside the body, or on a dry surface like a toilet seat. (So nobody is likely to get gonorrhea from a toilet seat, in spite of stories you hear.) But they grow rapidly on the warm, moist surfaces of the sex organs, and are spread from person to person during sex.

Signs and symptoms of gonorrhea. When a person has sex with someone who is infected, the gonococci make their way up into the urethra. There they begin infecting the cells lining these tubes. Uncomfortable symptoms begin between a day to a week after contact. In a boy, there is pain during urination and a thick, yellowish discharge from the penis. A girl may also have pain during urination, plus a yellow discharge from the vagina. This discharge usually increases in amount from day to day.

With this infection, there are no sores on the surface that you can see – one way to tell gonorrhea from genital herpes, where visible sores usually appear. With gonorrhea, the infection is internal. But a simple lab test can often show that the infection is there. A drop of discharge from the penis or vagina is put on a glass slide and stained. Then it is examined under the microscope. The slide will show many pairs of gonococci, colored bright red, along with many pus cells (dead white blood cells).

Although the first symptoms of gonorrhea are messy and uncomfortable, they aren't terribly painful. They may even be harder for a girl to notice than a boy. Sometimes people just pretend they aren't there. This is too bad, because this early stage of infection is the best time to treat and cure gonorrhea, before it has a chance to do serious damage. This is also a time when gonorrhea is *extremely contagious.* Any sex contact at this time is almost certain to spread the disease to others. If gonorrhea is discovered and treated at this early stage, it can be cured quickly. But if the infection isn't discovered, or is ignored, serious complications can result.

Complications of gonorrhea. One thing that can happen is that the germs, after growing and multiplying in the sex organs for a while, can get into the bloodstream and travel to the joints. There they can lodge and grow, causing a painful and damaging joint infection called *septic arthritis.* The knees are most frequently attacked, but the elbows or other joints can also be infected. Treatment can stop the infection at this point too. But long-term damage to the joints may occur if treatment is delayed.

In a girl, untreated gonorrhea can cause another kind of long-term trouble. After a few days or weeks, the early infection may seem to quiet down, even without treatment. But it isn't gone. During this time, the germs can work their way up into the Fallopian tubes and start an infection there. This can cause fever and severe pain in the lower abdomen. As the girl's body tries to fight the infection, the tubes become swollen and filled with pus. Then the tubes can become scarred and blocked. Doctors call this pelvic inflammatory disease, or PID. (Other bacteria can also cause PID, but many of the worst cases are due to gonorrhea.) Sooner or later the body may fight off this infection, or it may be cured by antibiotic treatment. But the scarring and blocking of the tubes often can't heal. In many cases this can make a woman permanently *infertile* (unable to have babies).

Gonorrhea can also attack perfectly innocent victims. If a woman has gonorrhea when her baby is born, the germs can get into the baby's eyes and cause blindness. Doctors or nurses now put medicated drops or ointment into every baby's eyes as soon as it is born, in case the mother might have gonorrhea and not know it. These medicines kill any bacteria present. They have saved the sight of thousands of babies over the years.

Treatment of gonorrhea. Because gonorrhea can be so harmful, it is important to treat and cure it as soon as possible. And it can be cured – but not as easily as it used to be. When penicillin was first discovered, a single large shot would cure gonorrhea overnight in 99 percent of cases. But today many gonococci have become *resistant* to penicillin. Now doctors must often use other antibiotics for several days or even longer to cure gonorrhea. And then the person must be checked from time to time after treatment to be sure the infection is completely gone.

Of course it would be good news if a vaccine could be found to protect people from gonorrhea. But so far no such vaccine has been developed. The best protection we have today is *prevention*. We will talk about how to prevent gonorrhea and other STDs in Chapter 7.

Syphilis

Syphilis is a very old disease. It first made medical history in the 1500s, when it spread all over Europe in a terrible epidemic. In those days it was called the Great Pox to tell it from another dreadful disease, smallpox. Then, as now, syphilis was spread by having sex. But nobody knew where the disease started. Italian soldiers called it "the French disease" and French soldiers called it "the Spanish disease." Some people think it might have been carried to Europe from the New World by the Spanish conquistadors. To this day, nobody really knows.

We *do* know that syphilis still strikes frequently today. There were 27,000 new or "first-stage" cases of syphilis and 40,000 "late-stage" cases reported in the United States in 1986. And among STDs, syphilis is one of the most dangerous – far more so than gonorrhea.

Syphilis is so dangerous because it can do so much damage to the body if it isn't discovered early – and often it isn't. It's easy to miss the earliest signs of the infection, or mistake them for something else. But unless detected early, the germ of syphilis soon "goes underground" to distant parts of the body. There the infection can spread silently for years. It can slowly attack the brain, the spinal cord, the blood vessels, or other organs, causing terrible destruction or even death.

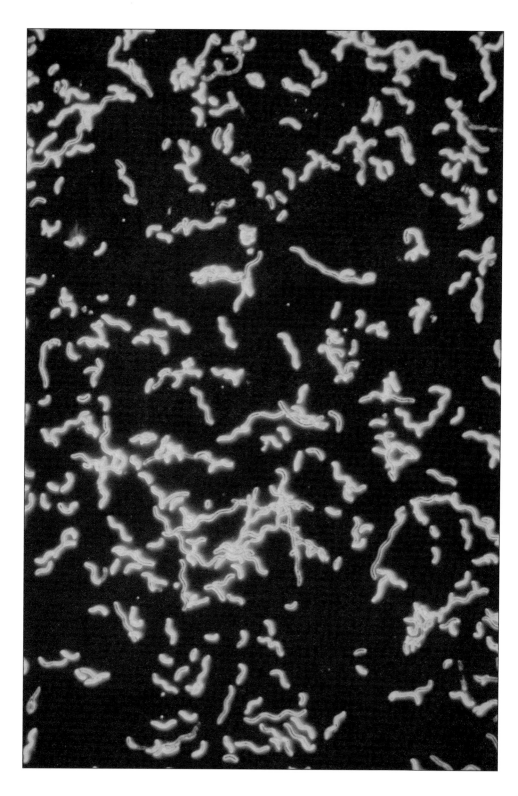

The first or primary stage of syphilis. Syphilis is caused by a tiny corkscrew-shaped germ called a spirochete. It is passed from one person to another during sex. This germ can burrow through the warm, moist surface of the penis or vulva and start growing just beneath the skin. The first sign of infection appears a week or more after contact. It is a small, painless sore called a *chancre* (pronounced SHANK-er). This usually forms somewhere on the sex organs. It may be on the penis, or the vulva, or even somewhere inside the vagina. Because it isn't painful, it can easily be missed. Even if noticed, it may be mistaken for genital herpes, except that it doesn't hurt the way genital herpes does. (See Chapter 5 for more about genital herpes.) Syphilis is very contagious – easily spread – at this stage, *primary syphilis*. As long as the chancre is there, it is teeming with spirochetes, so the infection can be passed on to anybody else the infected person has sex with.

This first sign of syphilis doesn't stay very long. The chancre seems to heal and go away all by itself in two or three weeks. But the infection is still there.

The second or secondary stage of syphilis. While the chancre is healing, the spirochetes have been multiplying rapidly and spreading to all parts of the body. Then, from one to six months later, a reddish-brown skin rash appears all over the body. This marks a second, more widespread stage of infection called *secondary syphilis*. During this stage, too, the infected person may be contagious and may pass the infection on to anyone by sexual contact. Soon, however, this rash also disappears, all by itself, as if it had never happened.

The third or tertiary stage of syphilis. However, the infection still hasn't gone away. It has just "gone underground" in the body. The spirochetes

Syphilis is caused by a corkscrew-shaped germ called a spirochete.

keep growing and multiplying, year after year, and begin causing harm to many of the internal organs. For years it may seem that nothing is happening. But sooner or later signs of this late-stage or *tertiary syphilis* begin to appear. The patient may suddenly have trouble walking because the spirochetes have destroyed nerve cells in the spinal cord. If brain cells have been destroyed, mental illness may begin. If blood vessels have been attacked by the spirochetes, they may weaken and burst. The heart, the liver, the bones, or any other organ may be ruined in this late stage of the infection.

How syphilis is detected. A person should suspect syphilis any time a sore appears on the sex organs (the primary stage of the infection) or an unexplained skin rash appears (the secondary stage of the infection). Either way, the infection can be detected if the spirochete can be seen under a microscope. Because this exam requires a very special microscope, and a lab technician who knows what the germ looks like, such an exam is usually done at an STD Clinic or Public Health Service laboratory.

In the primary *or first stage of syphilis, the spirochete germ invades the surface of the sex organs and causes a sore or* chancre. *In the* secondary *or second stage, after the chancre has healed, spirochetes invade the bloodstream and cause a reddish-brown skin rash. In the* tertiary *or third stage, months or years later, damage to the spinal cord, brain, arteries, or other organs will appear.*

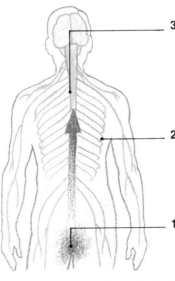

3. **The rash fades but the disease continues to attack the spinal cord and brain.**

2. **A reddish-brown skin rash appears on the body.**

1. **Spirochetes burrow into the sex organs causing chancre.**

Sometimes the germ just can't be found. Then another kind of test is useful. As soon as the spirochete enters the body, the body's immune system begins to fight against it. Special chemicals called **antibodies** appear in the blood to help destroy the germ. These "anti-syphilis" antibodies don't usually win – the infection keeps spreading in spite of them. But the antibodies stay in the blood as long as the germ is in the body. If a laboratory finds these antibodies in a sample of blood, that means the person has a hidden syphilis infection. In some states today this blood test must be done before a person can get a marriage license. Many hidden syphilis infections are discovered by this test.

Curing syphilis. Fortunately, most syphilis germs are killed very quickly by penicillin. Just one large dose of this drug may be all that is needed to cure the infection. But some people are allergic to penicillin. For them, other antibiotics will work just as well. Then, because this is such a dangerous infection, blood tests are done later to be certain the infection is gone.

Sometimes even innocent babies can fall victim to syphilis. If a woman with syphilis becomes pregnant, the spirochetes in her blood can infect her baby even before it's born. The child then has *congenital syphilis* at birth. Serious harm to its body may already have been done. For this reason, a blood test for syphilis is run the first time a woman sees a doctor about her pregnancy. If she has unsuspected syphilis, she will be treated immediately, to protect both her and her baby.

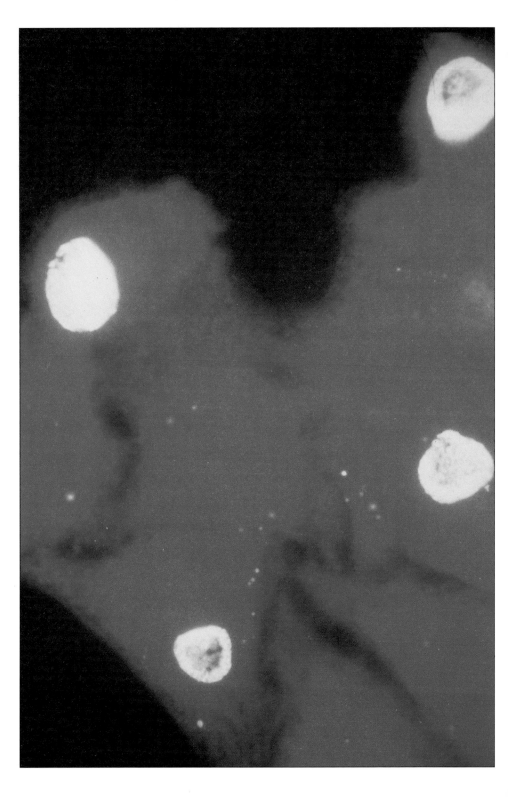

Chapter Four:
Chlamydia and Other STDs

Chlamydia is very hard to detect, and more than one lab test is needed to make sure it has been identified correctly. But once it is discovered and treated, it can be cured in one to three weeks.

Most people have heard about the danger of gonorrhea and syphilis. But there are some other STDs you may never have heard of at all. Some of them are uncommon in this country. But at least one – chlamydia, a major cause of infertility in women – may be more widespread than all the rest put together.

Chlamydia

Until ten years ago even doctors didn't know a lot about chlamydia. But today, some medical experts say it is the most widespread of all STDs. Certainly it is one of the hardest to detect.

Chlamydia (cluh-MID-ee-ah) infections are caused by tiny germs about halfway in size between small bacteria and large viruses. Similar germs cause *trachoma* (an eye infection that causes blindness) and *psittacosis*, or "parrot fever" (a kind of pneumonia people get from infected birds). The germ is so small it can't be seen under an ordinary microscope. This means other lab tests are needed to detect it.

Like all other STDs, chlamydia can infect both males and females. In males, the symptoms are a lot like those of gonorrhea. Two to three weeks after contact, there is pain and burning with urination, and a thin, whitish discharge from the penis. If a drop of this discharge is studied under the microscope and no gonorrhea germs are found, the doctor will suspect a chlamydia infection.

When any person has an STD, reinfection *can make successful treatment difficult or impossible. If one partner has an STD, both have it, and both should be treated. Unless both are treated at the same time, the one who isn't treated can reinfect the one receiving treatment and make cure impossible. This is one reason a person going to a doctor or clinic for treatment may be asked to identify any partners so they can be treated too. (Nobody is snooping or trying to get you in trouble.) Another reason is to help prevent wider spread of these diseases.*

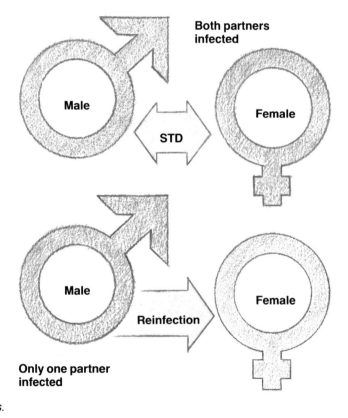

Both partners infected

Male

Female

STD

Male

Female

Reinfection

Only one partner infected

30

The situation is different in females. They may have no symptoms at all except a slight whitish vaginal discharge – no pain, burning, or other discomfort. This is because in females the chlamydia germ first infects the cervix, the lower end of the womb. If the girl or woman happens to have a *pelvic exam* (an examination of her sex organs) at this time, the doctor will see a sticky white discharge on her cervix. Laboratory tests would then reveal the infection. But with no symptoms, the woman may have no reason to see a doctor. This means that an early chlamydia infection is often overlooked.

Unfortunately, the infection doesn't go away. Untreated, it spreads up through the uterus into the Fallopian tubes. There it causes pelvic inflammatory disease much the same as the PID caused by gonorrhea. The tubes become infected, swollen, and scarred. If the woman becomes pregnant at this time, she is likely to have a dangerous *ectopic pregnancy*. (This is a pregnancy that starts growing in a tube instead of in the uterus where it belongs.) Later on, damage and blocking of the tubes may cause permanent infertility – inability to become pregnant. Some experts think that undiscovered chlamydia infections are largely responsible for the recent increase in the number of young women in their early 20s and 30s who can't get pregnant, no matter how hard they try.

Fortunately, the PID caused by chlamydia usually leads to symptoms – pain and cramping in the lower abdomen, for example, along with a mild fever. So a visit to a doctor or STD clinic at that time can lead to diagnosis and treatment.

Several different antibiotics can kill the chlamydia germ. Once the infection is discovered and treated, it can be cured in one to three weeks. But both the male and female partners need to be treated at the same time, if possible. This will prevent the kind of "back-and-forth" reinfection that often happens.

Trichomonas

A **trichomonas** infection is really more of a nuisance than a danger. This sexually transmitted infection (pronounced "trick-a-MO-nus") doesn't do any serious harm, except that it's very uncomfortable for girls and women. Like chlamydia, it is quite widespread. And because of the itching and burning it causes, it is sometimes confused with other STDs.

The germ, called *Trichomonas vaginalis*, lives and multiplies especially well in the vagina. It doesn't cause any blisters or sores. It just produces a thin, milky vaginal discharge that causes severe itching and burning. Since the germ is quite large, it can easily be seen under the microscope in a doctor's office or clinic. Once diagnosed, there are some simple medicines that will cure a trichomonas infection.

The treatment may not be permanent, however. For a long time "trich" was thought to be exclusively a female infection. Today we know that boys and men can have the infection too without having any symptoms. This means that sex partners can easily pass the infection back and forth. It doesn't do much good to treat and cure the woman alone, because she is likely to be reinfected the next time she has sex with her partner. To get rid of this nuisance, both partners need to be treated at the same time.

Three Bad Actors

Three other very unpleasant STDs should be mentioned here. They have special symptoms, and require a doctor's care when they appear.

One of these, known as **chancroid infection**, is caused by a bacillus that produces a large, painful sore on or near the sex organs of either males or females. Sometimes this sore is confused with genital herpes, but a doctor can tell the difference. Chancroid infection can be cured quickly and completely with antibiotics. But if left untreated, the infected sores can spread and cause a great deal of damage and scarring.

The second of these bad actors, **granuloma inguinale**, is caused by another bacillus. It is a slow-moving infection that spreads deep under the skin around the sex organs, causing painful lumps and swellings. This infection can also be cured by antibiotics, but takes longer to heal.

The third of these infections, known as **lymphogranuloma venereum**, or **LVG** for short, is caused by a close cousin to the germ that causes chlamydia. But it results in quite a different kind of infection. The germ invades glands in the groin or around the sex organs and causes very

The bacteria which cause chancroid infection.

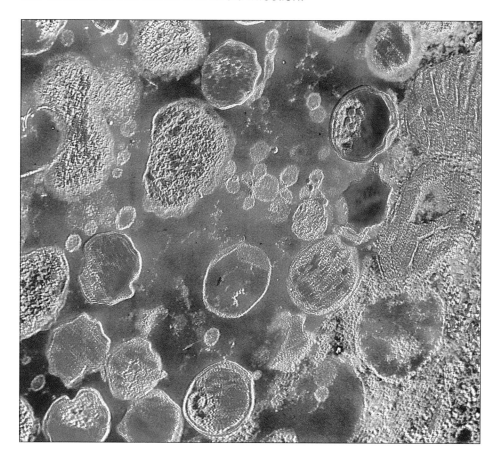

painful pus-filled swellings called **buboes**. This infection can be treated and cured with antibiotics.

These infections are not as common as gonorrhea or chlamydia, but they do turn up once in a while. The main message about them is that *anything* that causes painful sores, lumps, or swelling on or around the sex organs requires a doctor's attention. These infections will cause permanent damage and trouble only if you ignore the symptoms and don't get medical help.

Genital Warts

Genital warts are another common form of STD. They are wartlike growths that appear around the sex organs or the rectum. Genital warts are a lot like warts anywhere else on the body except that they grow quite large and are usually soft and moist. They are caused by germs known as **papilloma viruses**, usually passed from person to person by sex contact. There are chemicals that can get rid of them, or at least control them, by drying them up.

For a long while genital warts were thought to be just a nuisance. Recently, however, scientists have begun to think these wart-forming viruses may play a part in the development of cancer of the cervix in young women. For this reason, doctors today urge girls who develop these warts to have regular **Pap smears** – examinations for cancer of the cervix – beginning in their teenage years.

Hepatitis B

Hepatitis B virus attacks cells in the liver primarily. The disease is dangerous, with one out of ten victims dying from severe liver damage. But of those who recover, three out of ten continue to carry the live virus in their blood and body fluids, which means they can pass the infection on.

For a long while it was thought that the hepatitis B virus was only spread among drug users who shared dirty injection needles. But now we know that infected people also shed live viruses from moist body surfaces such as the sex organs. This means the infection can be passed on by sexual contact. So far there is no cure for hepatitis B. But there is a good vaccine to protect people at special risk (homosexuals, for example, or hospital workers, or family members of an infected person) from getting the infection.

Reading about these sexually transmitted infections may seem very unpleasant. All of them are disagreeable customers in one way or another. Some can cause serious trouble, and some are deadly. The one bright note in the picture is that all the STDs discussed so far (except hepatitis B) can at least be cured with antibiotics once they have been diagnosed.

Now we must look at two sexually transmitted diseases that can't be cured at all – and that's a different matter altogether.

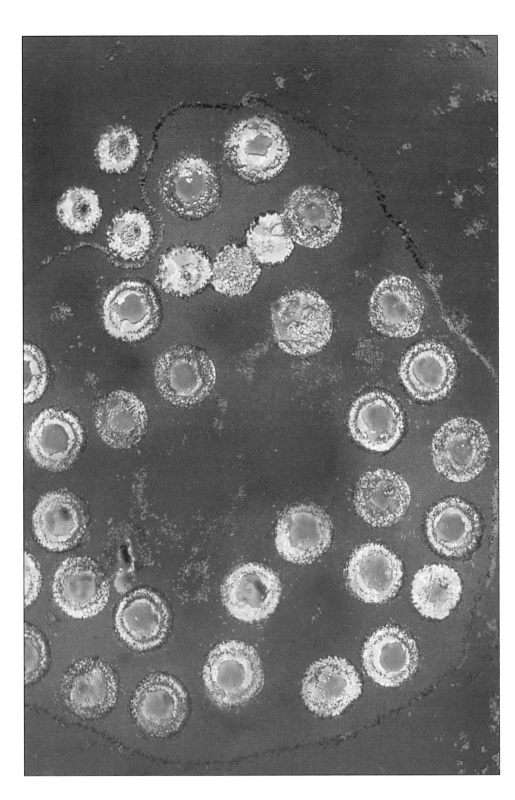

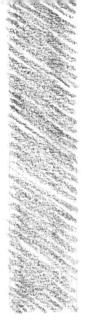

Chapter Five:
Genital Herpes

Genital herpes is one of the most widespread of all STDs today, particularly among young people. Although it doesn't usually kill anyone, it can't be cured and it doesn't go away.

Ten years ago, hardly anybody knew anything about genital herpes. That's not because it is a new infection. It's been around a long time, but until recently, it wasn't very widespread. Nobody talked about it. Even many doctors didn't know much about it.

All that has changed now. Today genital herpes is a full-fledged epidemic. It is spreading very fast, especially among teens and young adults. So it's important for young people everywhere to know some basic facts about this unpleasant infection:

1. It is a sexually transmitted disease. That means it is spread from person to person during sex.

2. It is one of the most widespread of all STDs today, particularly among teenagers and young people.

3. Though it doesn't usually kill anybody, or do dangerous things to the body, it *does* cause very unpleasant, painful symptoms.

4. Once a person has genital herpes, it can't be cured and it doesn't go away. It just hides in the body forever, causing new attacks of symptoms again and again, even after treatment.

The Genital Herpes Virus

Genital herpes (pronounced HER-pees) is caused by a virus called *herpes simplex virus 2*, or just HSV2. This is a germ so very tiny that it can only be seen with a special electron microscope. It is a close cousin to another virus called *herpes simplex virus 1*, or HSV1.

These two viruses invade the body through tiny scratches in the skin. Then they set up infections in the skin cells. HSV1 usually causes infections called *cold sores* on the lips or around the nose. But HSV2 invades the skin cells on or near the sex organs. Once inside those skin cells, HSV2 viruses force the skin cells to make more viruses very rapidly. These new viruses are then carried to the skin surface. From there they can be passed on to other people during sex.

First Symptoms of Genital Herpes

The first symptoms of genital herpes usually appear from two to seven days after having sex with someone who is infected. One or more clusters of small, red, itchy pimples appear on or around the sex organs. Most often they show up on the soft, moist folds of the vulva at the entry to the vagina, or on the skin of the penis. But they can also appear on the insides of the thighs, on the buttocks, or anywhere else in the area. For a few hours these pimples are just itchy. But soon they begin to ache and burn. Within a day or so the pimples change into painful clusters of fluid-filled blisters called *vesicles*. When these blisters break, they leave raw, painful, open sores.

At this point the infection is extremely contagious or "spreadable." This is because the open sores are teeming with new virus particles. Doctors would say that the infected person is "shedding virus." At this time the infection can easily be passed from one person to another by sexual contact.

This first or *primary* infection will last for about two weeks. Sometimes

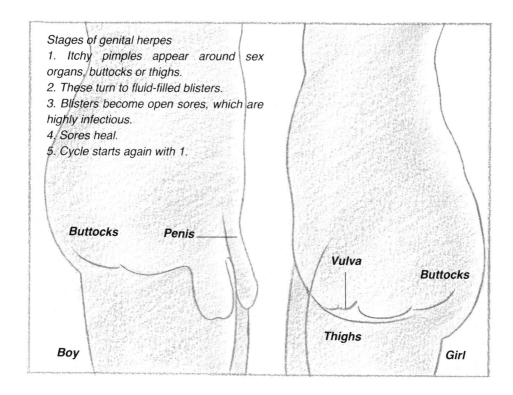

Stages of genital herpes
1. Itchy pimples appear around sex organs, buttocks or thighs.
2. These turn to fluid-filled blisters.
3. Blisters become open sores, which are highly infectious.
4. Sores heal.
5. Cycle starts again with 1.

Buttocks   Penis

Boy

Vulva

Buttocks

Thighs

Girl

other symptoms may occur as well. There may be a slight fever for the first two or three days, for example, or a vague feeling of being ill, or even some aching in the back, hips, or legs. These symptoms usually clear up in a day or so. Then, after about two weeks, the blisters and sores begin to heal too. After three or four weeks from the beginning of the primary infection, the active virus will be gone from the skin. The infected person will then most likely not pass the infection on to someone else during sex.

Recurring Infection

Just because the primary infection heals doesn't mean that the infection is over. Some lucky people – about 10 or 15 percent – never have any further trouble with genital herpes. But most people do. The HSV2 virus is temporarily gone from the skin – but it isn't gone from the body.

From the moment the HSV2 virus first invades the skin cells, the body's immune system starts making special antibodies to fight it off. But the virus isn't destroyed. It just runs and hides in nearby nerve cells, where the antibodies can't get at it. There it can stay "in hiding" for weeks or months – and then come back to cause another, or *recurrent*, infection. Some people have just one or two recurrent attacks. But others may have them again and again, several times a year. This can go on for years and years, whether the person is having sex or not. It's the same old infection coming back.

Recurrent attacks may not be quite as bad as the first one. The blisters appear again, usually in about the same places. But they may not hurt as much, and they often don't last as long – only a few days before healing. But these recurrent sores are the same as the first ones in one important way: they are shedding viruses again, so the infection can again be spread to others by sexual contact while they are present.

Genital herpes is not usually a deadly or damaging disease. It doesn't spread to other parts of the body. It doesn't attack a woman's tubes, as gonorrhea does, or destroy other organs, as syphilis can. For most people it is just a painful nuisance that comes back again and again. But there are special cases where it can be dangerous.

For example, if a pregnant woman has active genital herpes at the time her baby is due to be born, there is a chance the baby may contract the virus at the time of birth. Since the baby's immune system isn't very strong at that time, the child may develop a very severe infection – and some babies have died from this. For this reason, a pregnant woman with genital herpes must be observed very closely as delivery time nears. If her infection recurs and becomes active at the wrong time, it may be necessary

A baby can contract herpes at birth from its mother.

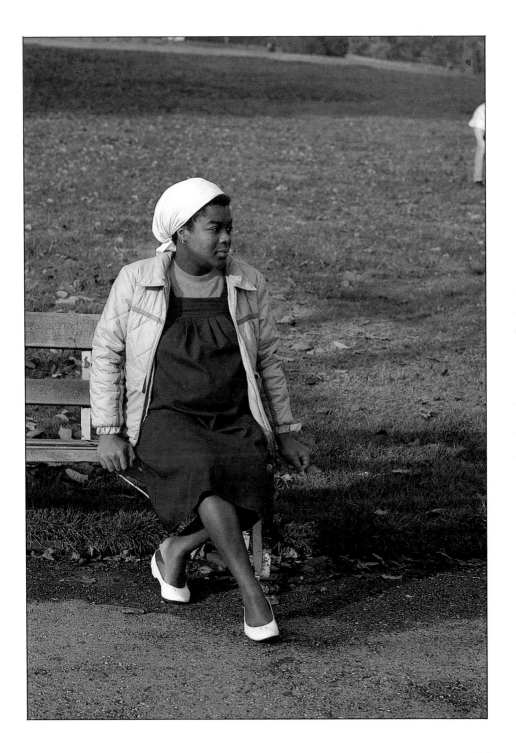

for her to have the baby by an operation called *cesarean section*, so that the baby doesn't contract the virus in the mother's vagina.

There is one other possible problem that scientists are investigating today. Doctors suspect that the HSV2 virus may make it easier for a woman to develop cancer of the cervix. This has not been proven yet. But we know that this kind of cancer sometimes appears especially early in women who have started sex at an early age, or had many different partners – women more likely to have been exposed to genital herpes. Fortunately, a lab test called a Pap smear can detect this cancer very early, when it is still completely curable. Any young woman who has genital herpes should have regular Pap smears to detect any sign of this cancer.

Treating Genital Herpes

Until about five years ago there was no good way to treat genital herpes. Once you were infected, there was nothing you could do about it. Then a drug called **acyclovir** (ace-EYE-clo-vir) was discovered. Acyclovir could prevent the HSV2 virus from reproducing itself in cells grown in the laboratory. When this drug was put in an ointment and rubbed on the active sores and blisters of genital herpes, they seemed to heal and become virus-free several days sooner than usual. Later, the same drug in pill form was given by mouth to people with severe, recurrent attacks of genital herpes. Many of those people then had fewer recurrences, and the attacks were shorter and less painful.

Acyclovir has to be ordered by a doctor. For many people with genital herpes, it will shorten the primary infection and reduce the frequency and pain of recurrent attacks. But it does *not* kill the virus or cure the disease. It just makes genital herpes a little easier to live with. Today other anti-virus drugs are also under study in hopes that a real cure for genital herpes may someday be found. And a search is on to find a vaccine that might protect

42

people from getting the infection in the first place. But so far, acyclovir is the best treatment there is.

Preventing Genital Herpes

Obviously, genital herpes is an extremely disagreeable infection to catch. Since it isn't curable, and doesn't go away once you've caught it, *preventing* it makes far more sense than taking the risk of catching it. In Chapter 7 we'll talk about the common-sense steps that anybody can take to keep from getting *any* kind of sexually transmitted disease. But since prevention is the *only* good answer to genital herpes, we need to preview some of those preventive steps right here.

1. *Saying "no" to sex* is the safest, surest way there is to keep from getting genital herpes. If you decide to say "no" to sex for the time being, you won't get this infection. (Forget what you may have heard about getting it from a toilet seat. It's *possible*, but let's be honest: that's not how people get genital herpes. Having sex is.)

2. If you do have sex, the fewer partners you have, the less risk you run of catching the infection. Having sex with just one other person – someone you're sure isn't infected – is the second best way to keep from getting infected yourself. This is just common sense.

3. If you do have sex, *talk* with your partner about genital herpes *before you have sex*. Why talk about it? Because *most people who have genital herpes know they have it.* After all, the symptoms are hard to miss. Even if a person doesn't know for sure what's *causing* certain symptoms, he or she knows that *something* is wrong. There's no excuse for hiding it. If there's *any* possibility that either you or your partner might have genital herpes (or any other STD), sex should be postponed until a doctor can determine what's going on and what isn't.

4. If you do have sex, be sure to use a latex rubber **condom** (sometimes called a "rubber" or a "safety") to protect yourself. If you're a girl or woman, insist that your partner use one. *The genital herpes virus cannot get through a latex condom.* So using a condom whenever you have sex – and using it *properly* – will protect you from this infection. (But make sure it is latex rubber – a "natural" or "lambskin" condom won't protect you.) There are some simple rules for using condoms properly in Chapter 7.

Disagreeable as it is, you can live with genital herpes. But AIDS – another sexually transmitted disease – kills people. In the next chapter we'll check some basic facts you need to know about this deadly disease.

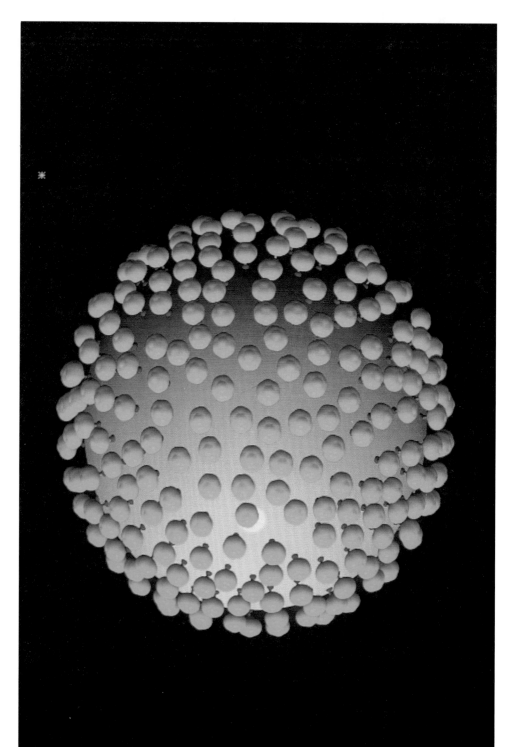

Chapter Six:
AIDS

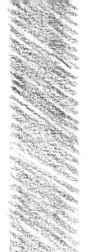

The worst sexually transmitted disease by far is AIDS, caused by the virus HIV. People who contract AIDS die of the disease – in most cases within about two years.

Any STD can mean trouble for the person who is infected. But of all the sexually transmitted diseases we know about, AIDS is by far the worst. AIDS kills people. It is one of the most deadly infections ever known. It is also an infection that is spreading rapidly today. It is a terrible threat to everbody, including young people who are sexually active.

For this reason, everybody needs to know some hard facts about AIDS. What is it? What can it do to you? How can it be spread from person to person? And above all, how can you protect yourself from it?

A New and Deadly Virus

Unlike other STDs, which have been around for many years, AIDS is a newcomer. The first cases were found in the United States as recently as 1981, although some unrecognized cases may have occurred much earlier. Since 1981, however, more than 70,000 people in the United States alone have become terribly ill from AIDS. Over 39,000 of them have already died. Many other cases and deaths have occurred worldwide. And scientists believe that more than one and a half million people in this country may already be infected with the deadly AIDS virus .

AIDS is caused by a tiny but deady **virus** which can cause terrible damage once it gets into a person's body. First this germ hunts out special blood cells called *lymphocytes* and works its way inside them. There the virus takes command of these cells and forces them to begin making more AIDS viruses. This process kills the lymphocyte cells, while the new viruses are released into the bloodstream. From there they go on to infect more lymphocytes.

Gradually, more and more lymphocyte cells are killed and more and more AIDS viruses are made. All this may take from a few months to eight or nine years without any actual symptoms appearing. Meanwhile, many AIDS viruses are present in the bloodstream and in other body fluids, particularly in a male's **semen** (the fluid he ejaculates during sex) and in a female's vaginal secretions.

Testing for the AIDS Virus
There may be no sign of infection for months or even years after the AIDS virus gets into the body. But there's a way to tell that the virus is there, just the same. Weeks to months after the virus first invades the body, the body's *immune protective system* discovers that it's there and goes into battle against it. Lymphocyte cells in the immune system start making special chemicals called antibodies to fight the viruses. These antibodies don't seem to kill the invading germs, but they hold them in check for a while. Meanwhile, by doing special blood tests, laboratories can detect the antibodies in the person's bloodstream. If the antibodies are there, it means the person is already infected with the AIDS virus, even though no symptoms of sickness have appeared. And if the AIDS virus is there in a person's body, that person can pass it on to others, whether he or she seems to be sick or not.

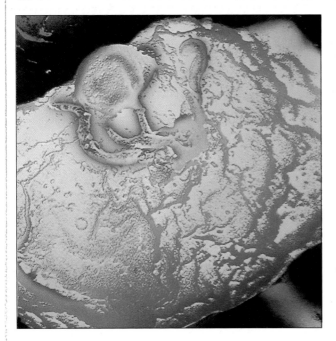

On entering the body, the AIDS virus HIV contacts a T-cell lymphocyte and injects its RNA genetic code into the cell. A virus enzyme called reverse transcriptase *splices the virus RNA into the T-cell DNA molecule. The T-cell is then forced to* replicate, *or duplicate, more HIV virus units and release them into the bloodstream. The T-cell is killed in the process. The drug AZT may help block or interfere with this virus-making process.*

How HIV multiplies

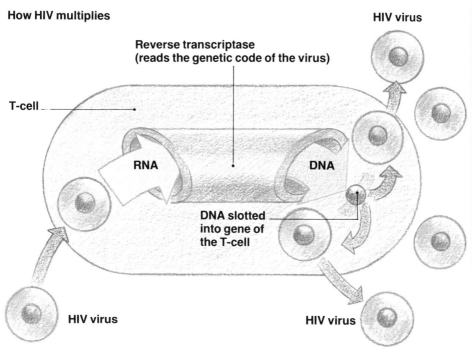

HIV virus

Reverse transcriptase
(reads the genetic code of the virus)

T-cell

RNA

DNA

DNA slotted
into gene of
the T-cell

HIV virus

HIV virus

Nobody can say exactly how long it will take a person to become sick from the AIDS virus once infected. Some people start getting sick within a few months. Others may not get sick for three or four years or even longer. Some may never get sick. Nobody knows for sure who will and who won't. But so far, about 30 percent of the people infected with the AIDS virus seem to get sick from it sooner or later. And once symptoms begin, there is little chance of recovery.

What AIDS Can Do

What exactly does the AIDS virus do to the body that's so bad? We know that the virus begins killing lymphocyte cells right from the start as new virus particles are made. But there's more to it than that. Lymphocytes are an important part of the body's immune protective system – the body's natural way of fighting foreign invaders like bacteria and viruses. One group of lymphocytes, called **B-cells**, make the antibodies that fight infectious germs. Another group, known as **T-cells**, help the B-cells make more antibodies faster in times of crisis. These are sometimes called "helper cells." The trouble with the AIDS virus is that it attacks and kills more of these particular T-cells or "helper cells" faster than any other kind of lymphocyte. As more and more of these "helper cells" are killed by the virus, the body's ability to make antibodies against disease germs is damaged more and more. After a while the body's immune defense system becomes so crippled or *deficient* that it can't do its job anymore – it's just wiped out. This is where the name "AIDS" comes from. It stands for *A*cquired *I*mmune *D*eficiency *S*yndrome. That means the disease is a *syndrome* (a group of bad symptoms) that has been caught or *acquired* (from a bad virus) that causes a *deficiency* of the body's *immune* system.

One of the symptoms of AIDS is extreme weight loss.

Symptoms of AIDS

What does all this mean? Without immune protection, the person with AIDS can begin coming down with a number of bad symptoms. Some start having nausea, vomiting, and extreme weight loss, or have high fevers and sweating at night. Others develop swollen glands all over the body.

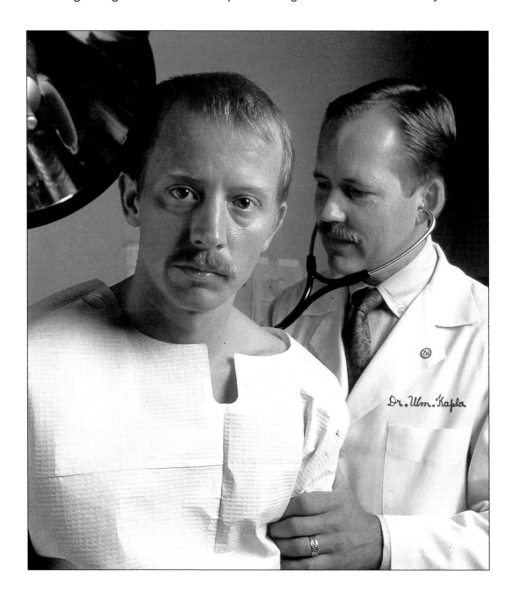

Still others have even more dangerous symptoms. There are many diseases normal people never get because their immune systems fight them down. But these diseases become deadly threats to people with AIDS who have lost their immune protection. Many AIDS patients, for example, come down with a deadly lung infection which is very hard to cure and keeps coming back. Others develop an unusual kind of cancer, seldom seen in normal people. And many people with AIDS have another kind of problem too. The virus may attack nerve cells as well as lymphocytes, causing severe problems with the way the brain and nervous system work.

These symptoms of AIDS may vary from person to person, but the final deadly nature of this disease is the same for everyone. Once symptoms

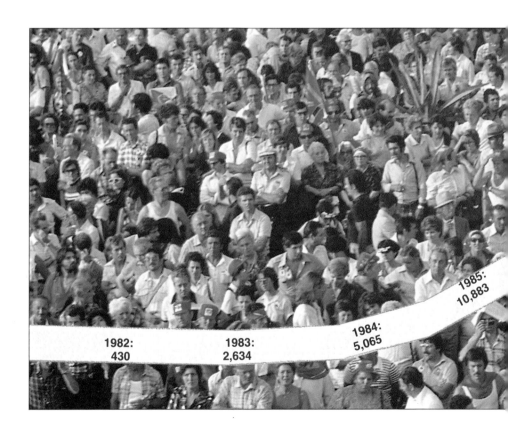

1982:
430

1983:
2,634

1984:
5,065

1985:
10,883

begin, the AIDS patient will die of the disease, usually within about two years. True, one drug recently discovered may help extend an AIDS patient's life for a while. But there is no *cure* for AIDS and no vaccine yet to protect against it. A person's only real protection is *not to become infected in the first place*. But to protect yourself you need to know how the infection is spread.

This graph shows the number of new *cases of AIDS diagnosed in the United States each year since 1982. These figures are for people with full-blown AIDS – the number of HIV carriers is much higher.*

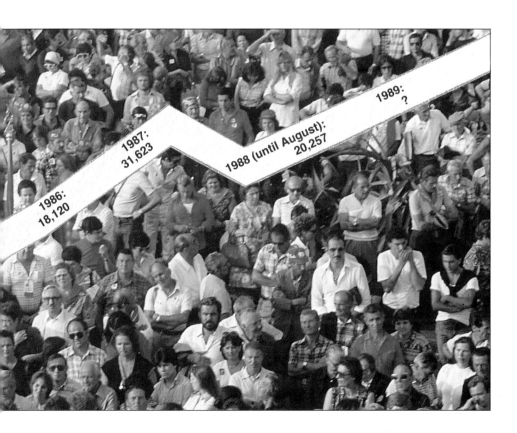

1986: 18,120

1987: 31,623

1988 (until August): 20,257

1989: ?

How AIDS Is Spread

When a person is infected by the AIDS virus, whether any symptoms have appeared or not, that person can pass the virus on to others. We know that the viruses are present in great numbers in the infected person's blood, in the man's semen, or the woman's vaginal secretions. It is contact with these fluids that can spread the AIDS virus. In fact, AIDS experts believe that AIDS is spread from person to person in just four main ways:

1. You can get AIDS by having sex with an infected person. This is the main route of infection for people who don't inject illegal drugs. *Any sex contact with an infected person is hazardous.*

Here we have to clear up a mistaken idea many people have about AIDS. Because so many of the first AIDS victims were male homosexuals (men who have sex with men), many people still think that AIDS is a "homosexual disease." They think that heterosexual people (those who have only male-female sex) are safe from infection. *This is not true. Anyone infected with the AIDS virus can pass it on to anyone else, male or female, during sex.* Many people in this country have already caught the infection from male-female contact, and in Africa and parts of Europe male-female sex is the main route of infection. In other words, *AIDS is a sexually transmitted disease.* And like any other STD, it can be passed on with *any* sexual contact with an infected person, homosexual or heterosexual.

Guarding Against AIDS

Once you know how AIDS is spread, you can see how to protect yourself from catching it.

For most young people, it's easy to avoid infected drug-injecting equipment. The rules are simple. *If you don't use illegal injectable drugs, never start. If you do use them, stop – for your life's sake.* And never use a needle for *anything* that somebody else has used for *anything.*

The connection between AIDS and dirty injection equipment is perfectly clear. Thousands of people have already gotten AIDS this way. But nobody *has* to use illegal injectable drugs, and it's possible for anyone using them to stop. If you are using them, *get help.* Talk to somebody – a doctor, a trusted counselor, your parents, a minister – *anybody you can trust* – to help you get out of a drug scene that could easily be deadly.

The risk of getting AIDS from sexual contact is harder to deal with. But

2. You can get AIDS by injecting drugs with dirty needles used by infected people. This is one of the most common ways that AIDS is transmitted in places like New York City, where there are large numbers of illegal drug users.

3. You can get AIDS by contact with contaminated blood or blood products. Before 1985, some people got AIDS from transfusions of infected blood. Many of them were people with a blood disease known as *hemophilia* who had to have frequent transfusions to stay alive. A number of school-age children got AIDS this way. Since 1985 all donated blood is tested for AIDS antibodies before it is used for transfusion, so this source of infection is very much reduced.

4. Finally, a woman infected with the AIDS virus can pass the virus on to infect her unborn baby. This accounts for hundreds of cases of AIDS in newborn babies.

It's important to know how AIDS is passed on from person to person. But it's also important to know how it *isn't* passed on. For instance, it *isn't* passed on by casual contact with an infected person in the classroom or on the playground. It *isn't* passed on by sneezing or coughing or noseblowing the way a cold or the flu might be. And it *isn't* passed on by using the same toilet facilities. The ordinary person going to school or work just doesn't have to worry about catching AIDS from casual contact. Basically, there are just two things you *do* have to worry about: catching AIDS from dirty drug-injecting equipment, or from sexual contact.

there are things you can do to protect yourself here, too. These same things will help protect you from *any* sexually transmitted disease, not just AIDS alone. Let's look at these things in detail in the next chapter.

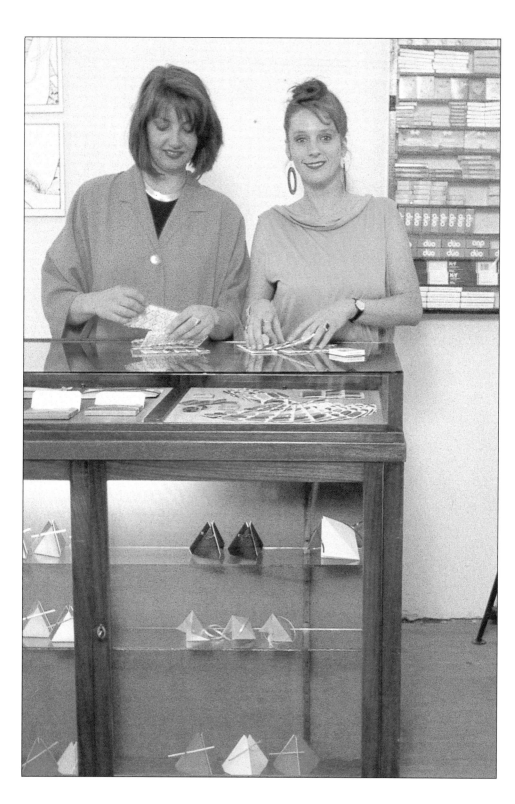

Chapter Seven:
Protecting Yourself Against STDs

STDs are easy enough to avoid. You have to be careful who you have sex with, and make sure you take a few simple precautions (like using a condom and spermicide) when you do choose to have sex.

A person reading this book might think that just about everybody has trouble with sexually transmitted diseases all the time. Of course that's not true. Many people spend their whole lives without ever once having an STD. People who pick their sexual partners very carefully – after long, close acquaintance – don't often get STDs. Neither do married couples who have sex exclusively with each other. They may worry about having unwanted pregnancies, but not about STDs.

Other people *do* risk getting these infections – some more than others. The ones who run the greatest risk are people who have lots of sexual contacts with lots of different people they don't know very well, or with people who are very likely to be infected, such as casual pick-ups or prostitutes.

Young people run a special risk of getting STDs for two reasons. First, they are just beginning to explore sex, without knowing too much about their partners, or even what STDs are all about. And second, there are already a lot of infected young people out there to catch these diseases from. In fact, the number of cases of sexually transmitted diseases today is increasing faster in young people in their teens than in any other age group.

Nobody *has* to get these infections. It is possible to keep from getting them at all. And if you do become infected, it is possible – in most cases – to get treatment before you suffer any bad consequences.

How can you protect yourself? Knowing what STDs are, and the problems they can cause, is a big step in the right direction. After that, protecting yourself depends on two things: *living defensively* and *getting medical help when you need it.*

Living Defensively

In King Arthur's time, when a knight rode out to battle, he wore his armor and shield, and carried his sword, dagger, and battleaxe along with him for protection. He knew there were nasty dragons out there who weren't interested in his safety. If he wanted to be protected from danger, he would have to do it himself, because nobody else was going to do it for him. He believed in *living defensively.*

Life is still a lot like that, as far as sexually transmitted infections are concerned. If you catch an STD, *you* are the one in trouble, nobody else. Maybe the person you have sex with will worry about protecting you, but you'd better not count on it. Like that knight riding out to battle, you need to be ready to protect yourself. "Living defensively" simply means arranging your life to protect yourself against these infections as much as is reasonably possible. Living defensively will offer you the *best possible protection against getting AIDS*, the terrible epidemic we talked about in the last chapter. But it can also protect you from all the other sexually transmitted diseases as well. Here are some pointers for living defensively:

1. *Say "no" to drugs.* We know that using dirty drug-injection equipment is a major way that AIDS is spread from person to person. Thousands of people have already gotten AIDS this way. Anybody who injects drugs is taking a tremendous risk. Hepatitis B, another dangerous infection, is also spread this way.

The rules for self-protection here are very simple. *If you don't use illegal injectable drugs, never start – not even once, just to "try it." If you do use them, stop – for your life's sake. And never, for any reason, use a needle or syringe that somebody else has used.*

As we mentioned in the last chapter, nobody *has* to start using injectable drugs, and those who do use them can stop. All kinds of people have done it.

2. *Say "no" to sex.* There are lots of reasons why having sex is pleasant and desirable. But sexually transmitted diseases are one very big reason why having sex may *not* be such a pleasant and desirable idea, at least for now. One of the facts of life is that young people who say "no" to sex, at least for the time being, don't have to worry about STDs.

Of course there are lots of other reasons today to consider postponing sex for a while. These could include your parents' concerns for you, your church's teachings, or your community's attitudes toward sex and marriage. Maybe the most important reason is your own sense of being your own person and making your own decisions. Lots of young people aren't all that eager to start having sex right away anyway. But some feel pressured into it by those around them. When you realize that STDs are a real threat, and that saying "no" to sex is the surest way to protect yourself against them, this knowledge may help you make (and stick to) a decision you'd just as soon make anyway.

3. *Keep self-protection in mind.* If you do have sex, make it a *monogamous*, or "one-person," relationship. It's just common sense that *the more different sex partners you have, the greater your risk of coming in contact with the AIDS virus or other STDs.* The fewer sex partners you have, the smaller the risk. And the better you know your sex partners, the less the risk. Best of all is to pick one partner you know hasn't had a lot of sex contacts previously, and then keep *your* sex relationship very much "one-person only."

4. *No matter how well you know your partner, use a condom and a spermicidal jelly or foam whenever you have sex.*

A **condom** (sometimes called a "rubber" or "safety") is a rubber tube, closed at one end, which is rolled down over a male's erect penis before he

1. *Use a condom every single time you have sex.*

2. *The boy should put on the condom as soon as his penis is erect, before he has any contact with the girl's vulva or vagina.*

3. *Squeeze the end of the condom between the fingers of one hand to keep the air out. Then roll the condom all the way down to the base of the penis before starting sex.*

4. *The boy should coat the condom with a spermicidal jelly or foam before sex. This will make the outside slippery and keep the condom from tearing.* Don't use vaseline or vegetable oil for this. *These things make the rubber break down.*

5. *The girl should put the spermicide into her vagina before sex, using the applicator that comes with the tube or can. This combination of spermicide and condom, used together, gives very good protection against STDs for both partners.*

6. *The boy should pull his penis out soon after climax, before it gets soft, holding onto the rim of the condom so it doesn't slip off. This will prevent any direct physical contact that might let STD germs pass*

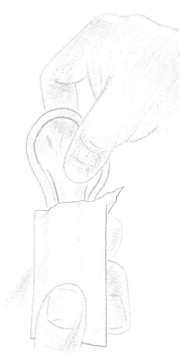

* Adapted from Hatcher, Robert. *Contraceptive Technology 1986-1987* ed. 13, New York: Irvington Publishers, 1987; and Goldsmith, Marsha F. "Medical News and Perspectives," *Journal of the American Medical Association*, May 1, 1987, Vol 257, No. 17.

starts having sex. The condom prevents actual direct contact between penis and vulva or vagina during sex. Scientists have shown that even a germ as tiny as the AIDS virus cannot get through an ordinary latex condom or rubber. Neither can the germs that cause gonorrhea, syphilis, genital herpes, or other STDs.

A **spermicide** is a jelly or foam that contains a chemical called *nonoxynol-9*. This chemical kills sperm cells on contact. It also kills many STD germs. So using a spermicide along with a condom adds extra protection against many STD germs.

For this condom-and-spermicide combination to really protect you against STDs, you have to use it correctly. Here are some "condom sense" rules to follow: *

from one person to the other.
7. Don't use the same condom more than once.
Using a condom and a spermicide is just another part of living defensively – protecting yourself – against contact with STDs until the time you and your partner are ready to establish a more permanent relationship.

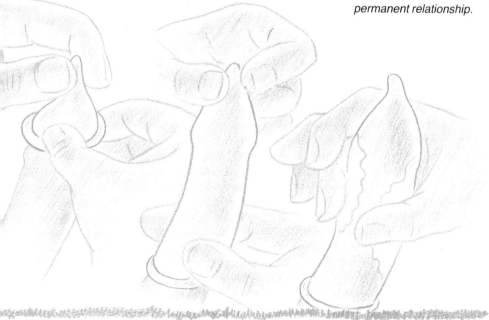

Glossary

AIDS (Acquired Immune Deficiency Syndrome) – a fatal infection, caused by a virus, which can be passed from one person to another during sex.

Acyclovir – a drug that helps prevent some viruses, like the genital herpes virus, from multiplying.

Antibodies – special chemicals the body makes to travel in the bloodstream and fight viruses and other foreign invaders.

B-cells – a group of lymphocytes (white blood cells) that help the body manufacture antibodies.

Body of the uterus – the upper, rounded part of the uterus, or womb.

Buboes – painful, pus-filled swellings around the groin or sex organs, caused by some STDs, especially LVG.

Cervix – the narrow lower end of the uterus, or womb, connected to the vagina.

Chancroid infection – an STD that produces a large, painful sore on or near the sex organs.

Chlamydia – a common STD that is especially dangerous to girls because it can infect their Fallopian tubes and prevent them from having babies later.

Condom – a thin latex rubber tube, closed at one end, that can be rolled down over the boy's penis before sex to help prevent STDs.

Erection – enlargement and stiffening of the boy's penis when he becomes excited about sex.

Fallopian tubes – the tubes that carry ripened egg cells from the girl's ovaries to her uterus.

Genital herpes – an STD, caused by a virus that produces outbreaks of painful sores on or around the sex organs.

Gonorrhea – one of the most common STDs, caused by a germ that attacks the urine tube or a girl's Fallopian tubes.

Granuloma inguinale – an STD, caused by bacillus, that produces painful swelling deep under the skin around the sex organs.

Infections – sicknesses that start when micro-organisms (germs) of various kinds get into the body. In *Sexually transmitted diseases* (STDs) the germs are passed from one person to another during sex.

Labia – the folds of a girl's external sex organs, just outside the opening of the vagina.

Lymphogranuloma venereum (LVG) – another STD that causes painful swellings around the sex organs.

Ovaries – the female sex glands which produce ripened egg cells ready to be fertilized by the male sperm.

Pap smear – a simple lab test, taken during a physical examination, to detect early signs of cancer in a woman's cervix.

Papilloma viruses – a family of viruses that can cause ordinary warts. They can also cause *genital warts* around the sex organs or rectum. Scientists today think they may help cause cancer of the cervix in women.

Pelvic inflammatory disease (PID) – an infection, usually sexually transmitted, that attacks a girl's Fallopian tubes or uterus. Most often due to gonorrhea or chlamydia infections.

Pelvis – the lowest part of the abdominal cavity, where the girl's internal sex organs (ovaries, Fallopian tubes, and uterus) are located.

Penis – the tube-shaped sex organ between the boy's legs.

Protozoans – tiny, single-celled, animal-like micro-organisms which sometimes cause infection when they get into the body.

Scrotum – the small sack behind the boy's penis which holds the male sex glands or testicles where sperm cells are made.

Semen – the fluid, containing sperm cells, that comes out of the boy's penis when he *ejaculates*, or comes, at the end of sex.

Spermicide – a chemical, usually in a cream or jelly, that kills sperm cells on contact.

Syphilis – an ancient and deadly STD caused by a germ called a *spirochete*. In the first or primary stage of infection the spirochete causes an open sore on or near the sex organs. In the secondary stage the germ spreads into the bloodstream, causing a rash all over the body. In the third or tertiary stage the germ attacks and destroys many body organs including the nervous system, and finally causes death.

T-cells – a group of lymphocytes (white blood cells) that help control how fast or slow the B-cells make antibodies to fight an infection. T-cells are the particular cells killed by the AIDS virus, damaging the body's immune defense system.

Testicles – the male sex glands, which produce sperm cells.

Trichomonas – an infection, caused by a protozoan micro-organism, that produces troublesome itching and discharge from the vagina.

Urethra – the urine tube which carries urine from the bladder to the outside.

Uterus – the organ, commonly called the *womb*, in which the new baby grows when a girl becomes pregnant.

Vagina – the tube, leading from the girl's external sex organs to her cervix, where the boy inserts his penis during sex.

Viruses – the smallest of the germs that can cause infections when they get inside the body.

Vulva – a girl's external sex organs, including the labia and the entrance to the vagina.

Yeasts – a form of fungus that can cause certain infections in the body.

Index

Photographic Credits
pages 4 and 54: Rex Features; pages 10,
12, 14, 18, 24, 28, 33, 37, 42, 44, 47 and
49: Science Photo Library; page 50: Zefa.,